Keto Dinner Cookbook for Women Over 50

Quick and Easy Recipes to Stay Fit and Lose Weight Fast

Katie Attanasio

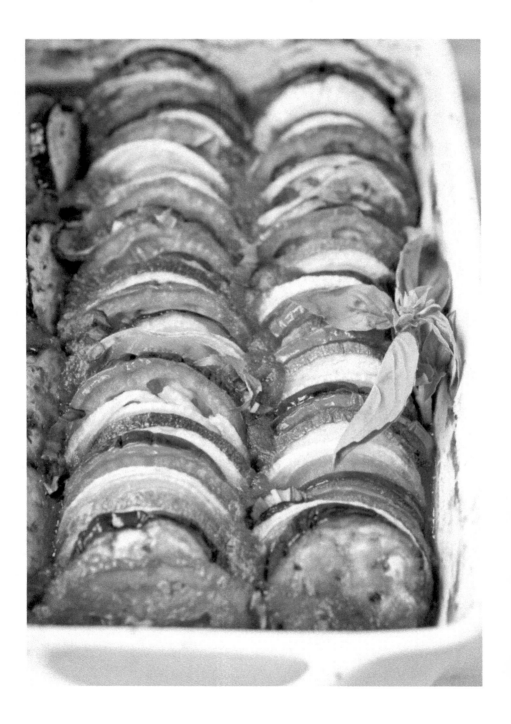

Table of Contents

50 Keto Dinner Recipes

1   Keto Shepherd's Pie

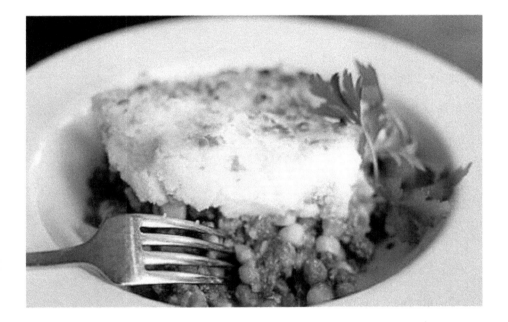

Servings: 6 | **Time**: 1 hr. 30 mins | **Difficulty**: Difficult

Nutrients per serving: Calories: 476 kcal | Fat: 37g | Carbohydrates: 10g | Protein: 26g | Fiber: 3g

Ingredients

1 1/2 Lbs ground beef

2 Cups Water or Beef broth

One cubed Carrot

1/2 Cup chopped Onion

One cubed Turnip

1/2 Tsp Black pepper

2 Tsps Worcestershire Sauce

1 Tsp Beef Base

1 Tbsp Tomato paste

1 Tsp dried thyme

1 Tbsp Porcini powder dried

1/2 Tsp Salt

1/4 Tsp Xanthan gum

1/4 Cup chopped parsley

Mashed Cauliflower Topping

1/4 Cup Sour cream

1 Lb tendered cauliflower florets

1/2 Cup sliced Scallion tops

2 oz soft Cream cheese

1/4 Tsp Salt

1 Cup grated Gruyere Cheese

¼ Tsp white pepper

Method

1.   Collect and prepare all the ingredients.

2.   Mix xanthan hum and spices in a bowl. Try not to form clumps.

Cottage Pie Filling:

1.   Cook ground beef in a pan over medium flame and use a spoon to break it while cooking and stirring.

2.   Increase the flame and stir in veggies, Worcestershire, mixed spices, water, beef base, and tomato paste.

3.   Mix well to dissolve tomato paste and beef base.

4.   Cover the pan and let it simmer for 22 minutes over a low flame or until veggies are done.

5.   After 20 minutes, increase the flame and let the gravy to get a thicker consistency.

6.   Sprinkle parsley and add salt and pepper to adjust the taste. Mashed Cauliflower Topping

1.   Place cauliflower in a bowl and add a little water.

2.   Place the bowl in the microwave and let it steam for ten minutes with occasional stirring.

3.   Transfer the tender cauliflower to a blender and blend it.

4.   Pour in sour cream, pepper, cream cheese, and salt and blend again to get a smooth mixture.

5.   Shift the cauliflower mixture in a container and mix in cheese and scallion.

6.   Spread shepherd's pie filling in casserole sprayed with oil and add cauliflower mixture over it.

7.   Sprinkle cheese over the tip.

8.   Bake in a preheated oven at 375 degrees for 50 minutes.

9.   Serve and enjoy it.

2   Keto Lasagna Stuffed Peppers

Servings: 6 | **Time**: 1 hr | **Difficulty:** Difficult

Nutrients per serving: Calories: 660 kcal | Fat: 20g | Carbohydrates: 9.92g | Protein: 26.63g | Fiber: 1.3g

Ingredients

1 Cup ricotta cheese

3 Bell peppers

1/4 Tsp Fennel seeds

1 Tsp Olive oil

1 Lb ground Beef

1 1/2 Cup shredded Mozzarella cheese

1 Cup Tomato sauce

1/4 Cup Parmesan cheese

Method

1.   First, cut the peppers in half and deseed them.

2.   Place the deseeded bell peppers in a baking tray.

3.   Heat olive oil in a skillet over medium flame.

4.   Sauté fennel seeds in heated oil with constant stirring.

5.   Add ground beef and cook while breaking it with the spoon.

6.   Add tomato sauce and cook for few minutes or when the sauce gets thickened.

7.   Now, remove the skillet from the flame.

8.   Add mozzarella cheese and set aside for a while. The meat sauce is ready.

9.   Then, fill the center of the bell peppers with meat sauce.

10.   Add ricotta cheese and again place a layer of meat sauce.

11.   Place the bell pepper in a baking tray and cover them with aluminum foil.

12.   Keep them aside for 25 minutes.

13.   Bake in a preheated oven at 350 degrees for 30 minutes.

14.   After 30 minutes, uncover the bell peppers, add mozzarella and ricotta cheese at the top and bake again for 12 minutes.

15.   Sprinkle parmesan cheese.

3 Herb Crusted Eye Round Roast Beef

Servings: 12 | **Time:** 1 hr 50 mins | **Difficulty**: Difficult

Nutrients per serving: Calories: 348 kcal | Fat: 15.37g | Carbohydrates: 1.91g | Protein: 47.63g | Fiber: 0.4g

Ingredients

1/4 Cup Dijon mustard

4 Lb eye round roast

Salt to taste

2 Tbsps Olive oil

Black pepper to taste

1/2 Cup crushed pork rinds

1/4 Cup minced Shallots

2 Tbsps minced Parsley

1/4 Tsp Pepper

1/2 Cup grated Parmesan Cheese

1/4 Cup Butter

2 Tbsps minced Garlic

1 Tbsp chopped Thyme

1/4 Tsp Salt

Method

1.   Combine minced shallots, herbs, parmesan cheese, pepper, garlic, and salt in a mixing bowl.

2.   Add pork rinds and toss well. Keep it aside for a few minutes.

3.   Rub roast with salt, olive oil, and pepper and set aside for few minutes.

4.   Heat olive oil in a pan with a heavy bottom.

5.   Add roast and cook from all sides until they turned brown.

6.   Transfer them to a plate and set them aside.

7.   Sprinkle Dijon mustard over the roast.

8.   Heat butter in the same pan and add all the ingredients of herb crust, and stir well.

9.   Lightly coat the roast with the herb mixture by pressing the mixture over it.

10.   Bake the roast in a preheated oven at 275 degrees until the roast's internal temperature reaches 135 degrees.

11.   Remove the roast pan from the oven and let it cool.

12.   Slice the roast with a sharp knife and serve.

4   Keto Korean Beef Bowls

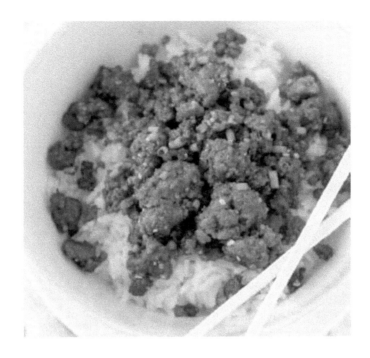

Servings: 2 | **Time:** 15 mins | **Difficulty:** Easy

Nutrients per serving: Calories: 462 kcal | Fat: 25.25g | Carbohydrates: 7.48g | Protein: 48.83g | Fiber: 2.5g

Ingredients

1 Tbsp Sesame oil

1 Tsp Ground Ginger

1 Lb Lean Ground Beef

1 pressed Garlic clove

2 Tbsps Tamari Soy Sauce

1/4 Tsp Chile flakes

1 Tbsp brown sugar

1 Tbsp Siracha

1 Tbsp White vinegar

1 1/2 Cups Cauliflower rice

1 Tbsp lime juice

Method

1.   Heat sesame oil in a skillet over medium flame.

2.   Add beef and stir well.

3.   Cook while stirring and break it using a spoon.

4.   Let it cook for five minutes until beef turned brown and no pink color is seen.

5.   Stir in garlic, chili flakes, and ginger.

6.   Increase the flame to high and cook for five minutes.

7.   Add soy sauce, sriracha, vinegar, and sugar.

8.   Cook for two minutes with constant stirring to evenly mix everything well.

9.   Remove the skillet from flame and mix in lime juice.

10.   Serve and enjoy it with cauliflower.

5 Keto Keema Curry

Servings: 2 | **Time**: 30 mins | **Difficulty**: Medium

Nutrients per serving: Calories: 268 kcal | Fat: 14.6g | Carbohydrates: 9g | Protein: 25g | Fiber: 3.3g

Ingredients

1 Lb ground Beef

3/4 Cup diced Onion

1 Cup sliced green Beans

One sprig Cilantro

1 Tbsp minced garlic

1 Tbsp Ghee

1 Tbsp minced Ginger

1 Tbsp Coconut Manna

3/4 Cup Water

1 Tsp ground Coriander

1/4 Tsp Red pepper flakes

1 Tsp ground Cinnamon

3/4 Tsp Salt

1/4 Tsp Turmeric

1/4 Tsp Black pepper

1/4 Tsp Fennel seeds

Three whole Green cardamon pods

Four whole Cloves

2 Tbsp Poppy seeds

Thin plain yogurt

Chopped Cilantro

Lime wedges

Method

1.   First ground fennel, poppy seeds, cloves, and cardamom in mortar and pestle and transfer them to a bowl. Set aside.

2.   Heat olive oil in a skillet over medium flame.

3.   Sauté onions in heated oil for six minutes.

4.   Stir in ginger and garlic and cook for one minute.

5.   Mix in ground beef and, using a spoon breaking it and cook until it turned brown.

6.   Bow pour in coconut mana or coconut milk, whatever you are using.

7.   Add spices and mix well—Cook for two minutes.

8.   Add green beans, water, and cilantro.

9.   Cover the pan and let simmer for 15 minutes, until beans are done.

10.   Sprinkle salt and pepper to adjust the taste.

11.   Sprinkle cilantro and lime. Pour in the yogurt and serve

6   Tofu Lettuce Wraps

Servings: 2 | **Time**: 20 mins | **Difficulty**: Easy

Nutrients per serving (4 wraps): Calories: 338 kcal | Fat: 28.3g | Carbohydrates: 7.8g | Protein: 17.7g | Fiber: 3g

Ingredients

2 Tsps Sesame Oil

12 oz Firm Tofu

One thumb-sized Ginger

2 Green Onions

Eight leaves of Baby Gem Lettuce

For the Peanut Sauce:

1 Tbsp Peanut Butter smooth

1 Tsp Rice Vinegar

1 Tbsp Sesame Oil

1 Tbsp Soy Sauce

1 Tbsp Water

Method

1.   Whisk all the items of peanut sauce in a bowl and keep it aside until further use.

2.   Heat sesame oil in a skillet over medium flame.

3.   Sauté onions and ginger in heated oil for three minutes.

4.   Now add chopped tofu and cook for six more minutes with frequent stirring.

5.   Pour in peanut sauce and toss well to coat everything in.

6.   Remove the pan from the flame and let it cool for a few minutes.

7.   Spread tofu mixture over a lettuce leaf.

8.   Sprinkle onions and sesame seeds.

9.   Serve and enjoy with peanut sauce as dipping.

7   Cajun Shrimp and Avocado Chaffle

Servings: 4 sandwiches | **Time:** 25 mins | **Difficulty:** Medium

Nutrients per serving: Calories: 488 kcal | Fat: 32.22g | Carbohydrates: 6.01g | Protein: 47.59g | Fiber: 2.6g

Ingredients

Cajun Flavored Chaffle:

4 Eggs

2 Cups shredded Mozzarella cheese

1 Tsp Cajun Seasoning

Chaffle Sandwich Filling:

1 Lb Raw Shrimp

4 Slices cooked Bacon

1 Tbsp Bacon fat

One sliced Avocado

One recipe Bacon Scallion

Cream Cheese Spread

1/4 Cup sliced Red onion

Method

1.   Whisk eggs in a bowl.

2.   Mix in mozzarella cheese and Cajun seasoning. Toss to evenly mix everything.

3.   Now transfer the batter to the waffle maker in batches and cook until they turned to brown.

4.   Combine shrimp, Cajun seasoning, pepper, and salt in a bowl.

5.   Heat bacon fat in skillet over medium flame.

6.   Add shrimps and cook until they get opaque for five minutes from both sides.

7.   Transfer the cooked shrimps to a plate and keep it aside.

8.   Put some cream cheese over the chaffle, add shrimps, avocado, onion, and bacon.

9.   Place another chaffle over the first one.

10.   Serve and enjoy it.

8   Grilled Tandoori Chicken

Servings: 12 | **Time**: 50 mins | **Difficulty**: Medium

Nutrients per serving: Calories: 220 kcal | Fat: 9.7g | Carbohydrates: 0.8g | Protein: 29.4g | Fiber: 0.3g

Ingredients

For the Grilled Tandoori Chicken Marinade:

2 Tbsp Garam Masala

1 Tsp Turmeric

1 Tbsp Paprika

1/4 Cup Water

¼ Tsp Cayenne Chili Powder

1 Tsp minced Garlic

1 Tsp minced Ginger

3 Tbsp Olive Oil

2 Tbsp Lime Juice

Method

For the Marinade:

1.   Whisk all the ingredients of marination in a bowl except for lime juice and water.

2.   A smooth paste is formed.

3.   Now mix in water and lime juice and adjust the consistency.

4.   Add the chicken and toss well to thoroughly coat the chicken.

5.   Cover the bowl and place it in the fridge for five hours to marinate the chicken.

Grilled Tandoori Chicken:

1.   Place the marinated chicken without marinade over the preheated grill.

2.   Cook for five minutes while covering the grill.

3.   Change the side of the chicken and cook for another three minutes.

4.   Repeat the process and continue it for 15 minutes until the whole chicken is fully tenderized.

5.   Serve and enjoy it.

9   Keto Chicken Stuffed Peppers

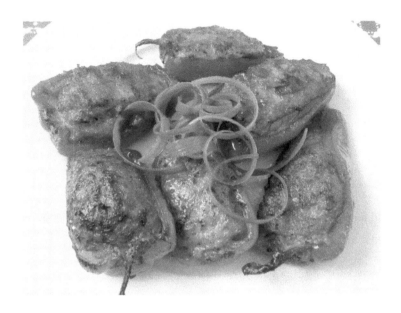

Servings: 4 | **Time**: 35 mins | **Difficulty:** Medium

Nutrients per serving: Calories: 468 kcal | Fat: 30g | Carbohydrates: 11g | Protein: 39g | Fiber: 2g

Ingredients

4 Bell peppers

2 Tbsps Olive oil

1/2 Tsp chopped Garlic

1 Lb ground chicken breast

One pinch of Salt

1 Tsp Pepper

1 Tbsp Lemon juice

1/2 Cup Pesto

1/4 Cup Parmesan cheese shredded

Four slices of Mozzarella cheese

Method

1.   Remove the seeds from bell peppers.

2.   Place deseeded bell peppers over a baking tray and bake in the preheated oven at 375 degrees for 15 minutes.

3.   Heat olive oil in a pan over medium flame.

4.   Add chopped bell peppers and cook for five minutes.

5.   When bell peppers get a little soft, add chicken breast pieces, salt, garlic, lemon juice, and pepper.

6.   Cook for few minutes with occasional stirring until chicken is turned golden.

7.   Drain the liquid released from the chicken and mix parmesan cheese and pesto.

8.   Toss everything well and remove the pan from the flame. The chicken filling is ready.

9.   Now take one baked bell pepper at a time and fill it with chicken filling.

10.   Drizzle mozzarella cheese and again bake for 18 minutes.

10   Egg Masala

Servings: 4 | **Time**: 30 mins | **Difficulty:** Medium

Nutrients per serving: Calories: 268 kcal | Fat: 21.8g | Carbohydrates: 8.7g | Protein: 11g | Fiber: 1.8g

Ingredients

Masala

Six hard-boiled eggs

¾ Cup chopped Onions

1 Lb chopped tomatoes

1/2 cup water

4 Tbsp Olive oil or ghee

Eight curry leaves

1-inch Cinnamon piece

One chopped Serrano pepper

Two chopped Garlic cloves

1 Tbsp Tomato paste

1 Tsp Chicken base

One sprig Cilantro

3/4 Tsp Coriander powder

Method

1.   Add all the ingredients of masala to a food processor and grind them to form a paste.

2.   Now add tomatoes without seeds in the processor and make a puree out of them.

3.   Add cinnamon and little water and blend.

4.   Transfer the puree to a bowl and set aside.

5.   Heat ghee in a pan over medium flame.

6.   Sauté curry leaves and cinnamon for 30 seconds.

7.   Now add onions and cook until they get brown color.

8.   Stir in masala mixture puree and cook until their raw smell goes off.

9.   Pour in a half cup of water and mix well.

10.   Cover the pan and let it simmer until everything is done.

11.   Add ghee, salt, and pepper, and toss well.

12.   Now mix in boil eggs and let them simmer for two minutes.

13.   Sprinkle cilantro and serve.

11   Juicy Keto Oven-Baked Ribs

Servings: 6 | **Time:** 3 hrs | **Difficulty**: Difficult

Nutrients per serving: Calories: 445 kcal | Fat: 32.5g | Carbohydrates: 3.39g | Protein: 37g | Fiber: 0.6g

Ingredients

2 Baby back ribs racks

2 Tbsps BBQ Dry Rub

Black pepper to taste

2 Tbsps Olive oil

Salt to taste

1/2 Cup Keto BBQ Sauce

Method

1.   First, remove the skin from the ribs using a sharp knife. Do it very carefully.

2.   Drizzle olive oil over the skinless dried ribs.

3.   Sprinkle salt and pepper over the ribs. Rub the seasoning to thoroughly coat the ribs.

4.   Place the ribs in a baking tray lined with aluminum foil and cover them.

5.   Bake in a preheated oven at 275 degrees for two hours or until ribs are fully tenderized.

For Keto Dry Ribs:

1.   Take the ribs out of the oven.

2.   Uncover the ribs and message them with salt and pepper again.

3.   Bake again for 22 more minutes without covering them. For Sauced Keto Ribs:

1.   Take the ribs out of the oven and remove the foil from them.

2.   Spread BBQ sauce over the ribs.

3.   Let them boil for five minutes over medium flame or until dark spots appears over the sauce.

4.   Repeat the process with the second side.

5.   Serve and enjoy it.

12   Indian Chicken Curry

Servings: 4 | **Time**: 40 mins | **Difficulty**: Medium

Nutrients per serving: Calories: 352 kcal | Fat: 24.5g | Carbohydrates: 5.7g | Protein: 29g | Fiber: 1.2g

Ingredients

Masala

1 1/4 Lb boneless Chicken breast

1/2 Cup sliced Onion

2 Tbsp Ghee

2 Tbsps Olive oil

1/4 Cup chopped cilantro

1/2 Cup Water

1/4 Tsp Salt

1 Tsp Chicken base

1/4 Tsp Turmeric

Two chopped Serrano peppers

3/4 inch chopped Ginger

One chopped green bell pepper

One chopped Garlic clove

Method

1.   Add all the ingredients of masala to the blender and blend them to form a paste. You can add a few drops of water too.

2.   Heat olive oil in a pan over medium heat.

3.   Add onions to heated oil and sauté them for three minutes.

4.   Stir in the masala paste and cook until their raw smell diminishes.

5.   Then add cinnamon, chicken base, turmeric, olive oil, and half Cup of water. Mix well.

6.   Now add chicken and toss well to mix everything.

7.   Cover the pan and cook for 15 minutes over low flame.

8.   After 15 minutes, remove the cover from the pan and increase the flame to evaporate all the water to thicken the chicken sauce.

9.   The oil will be seen over the sauce's surface, which indicates that the chicken is done.

10.   In the end, add ghee and sprinkle cilantro, and toss.

11.   Serve and enjoy it.

13 Stuffed Poblano Peppers with Mexican Ground Beef

Servings: 4 | **Time:** 50 mins | **Difficulty:** Medium

Nutrients per serving: Calories: 395 kcal | Fat: 23.6g | Carbohydrates: 11.6g | Protein: 35.6g | Fiber: 3.6g

Ingredients

4 Poblano peppers

1 Tbsp Olive oil

2 Tbsps minced Cilantro

1 Lb ground Beef

1/2 Cup Diced onion

2 Tbsps Tomato paste

Two chopped Garlic cloves

1 Tbsp ground Chile powder

 1 Cup Beef broth

Salt to taste

1 1/2 Tsp Ground cumin

One pinch of Cinnamon

1 1/2 Cup grated Monterey Jack Cheese

1 Cup cooked Cauliflower rice

Black pepper to taste

For Topping:

Salsa Cilantro

Pumpkin seeds Cheese

Lime wedges Sour cream

Method

1.   Arrange poblano pepper in a baking tray.

2.   Place the tray in the broiler and let them roast for minutes or until the pepper gets blacken.

3.   Transfer the roasted pepper onto the plate and cover. Keep it aside until further use.

4.   Heat olive oil in a skillet over medium flame.

5.   Sauté garlic and onion in heated oil for three minutes.

6.   Mix in ground beef and cook while breaking it using the spoon.

7.   When beef is cooked for ten minutes, mix in tomato paste, cinnamon, chili powder, beef broth, and cumin with constant stirring to combine everything.

8.   Let the mixture simmer until the liquid is reduced to half.

9.   Sprinkle salt, cilantro, and pepper.

10.   Now, peel the skin from roasted peppers and make a vertical slit at the top using a knife.

11.   Remove the seeds from the center of the pepper.

12.   Place the poblano peppers in a baking tray. Set aside.

13.   Mix in cheese and cauliflower rice with the beef mixture and toss to combine everything well.

14.   Fill the poblano pepper with the beef mixture.

15.   Sprinkle some of the cheese at the top.

16.   Bake the stuffed poblano peppers in a preheated oven at 350 degrees for 15 minutes.

17.   Squeeze time juice over the top and serve with salsa and green salad.

14 Cast Iron Sloppy Joe Casserole

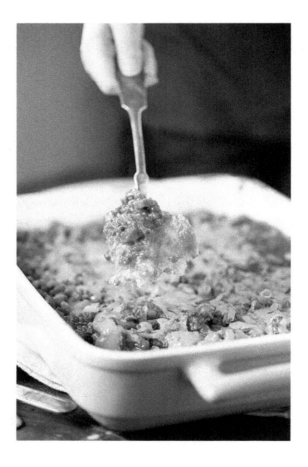

Servings: 8 | **Time:** 55 mins | **Difficulty:** Medium

Nutrients per serving: Calories: 371 kcal | Fat: 24g | Carbohydrates: 11g | Protein: 28g | Fiber: 3g

Ingredients

1 Cup Cheddar cheese

One recipe Sloppy Joes Cornbread Base

3 Eggs

1 Cup grated Mozzarella cheese

1/4 Tsp Sweet Corn Extract

2 oz Cream cheese

2 Cups Almond flour

1 Tbsp Baking powder

Method

1.   First, prepare the joe filling following the instruction written over the packet.

2.   Transfer the filling into the plate and sprinkle the cheese. Set aside until further use.

3.   Add extract, almond flour, cheese, baking powder, and eggs in a blender. Blend to get a thick batter.

4.   Transfer the batter into the bowl.

5.   Now spread the thick batter over a skillet sprayed with oil.

6.   Then, spread joe filling over the batter.

7.   Bake in a preheated oven at 350 degrees for 40 minutes.

8.   Again sprinkle cheese and bake to melt the cheese.

15   Slow Cooker Mississippi Pot Roast

Servings: 6 | **Time**: 6 hrs 20 mins | **Difficulty**: Difficult

Nutrients per serving: Calories: 503 kcal | Fat: 37.74g | Carbohydrates: 1.22g | Protein: 37g

Ingredients

2 1/2 Lbs Chuck roast

1/2 Tsp Salt

2 Tbsp Butter

1 Tbsp Olive oil

8 Pepperoncini peppers

1/2 Tsp Black pepper

1 Tsp Beef base

1/3 Cup Water

1 Tbsp Ranch Seasoning

Method

1.   Rub salt, oil, and pepper all over the surface of the chuck. Set aside until further use.

2.   Heat olive oil in a skillet over medium flame.

3. Add chuck roast and cook well from all the sides.

4. When the roast gets brown color, remove the skillet from the heat and transfer the roast to the slow cooker.

5. Now add beef base in the same skillet and cook over low flame.

6. Pour in water and let it simmer.

7. Transfer the beef base mixture into the slow cooker.

8. Add butter and ranch seasoning in a slow cooker and toss well.

9. In the end, add pepperoncini and cook for six hours on high flame.

10. When roast is done, transfer it to the plate.

11. Mix in 1 tsp of ranch seasoning and serve.

16 Lamb Chops with Mint Sauce and Roasted Rutabaga

Servings: 2 | **Time**: 50 mins | **Difficulty**: Medium

Nutrients per serving: Calories: 730 kcal | Fat: 56.7g | Carbohydrates: 10.23g | Protein: 39g | Fiber: 3.2g

Ingredients

Rutabagas

Mint Sauce

Four sliced Lamb loin chops

Salt to taste

2 Tsp Olive oil

Black pepper to taste

1/8 Tsp Salt

One cubed Rutabaga

2 Tsp Chopped Rosemary

2 Tsp Olive oil

1/8 Tsp Pepper

One pinch of Red chili flakes

1/4 Cup Champagne vinegar

1 Tbsp Minced Mint

2 Tbsp sugar One pinch of salt

Method

1.   Rub lamb with salt, olive oil, and pepper and set aside for a while.

2.   Add rutabaga, salt, olive oil, rosemary, and pepper in a bowl and toss to coat the rutabaga evenly.

3.   Transfer the rutabaga to a baking pan and cook with occasional stirring for about 32 minutes.

4.   Heat the olive oil in the same pan over medium flame.

5.   Add lamb chops and cook for 10 minutes from both sides.

6.   Shift the lamb chops into the plate and cover to keep it warm.

7.   In the same pan, add sweetener and vinegar.

8.   Let it simmer over low flame for seven minutes.

9.   Sprinkle salt, mint, and red chilies and toss well. The sauce is ready.

10.   Now cook rutabaga in the pan over medium flame for few minutes until it gets a golden color. Add salt and pepper and toss well.

11.   Transfer the rutabaga into the plate with cooked lamb.

12.   Pour the sauce over lamb and rutabaga and serve.

17 Ham Steak with Red-Eye Gravy

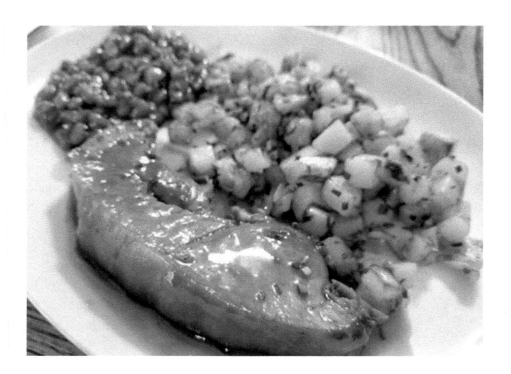

Servings: 4 | **Time**: 15 mins | **Difficulty**: Easy

Nutrients per serving: Calories: 417 kcal | Fat: 32g | Carbohydrates: 0.26g | Protein: 31g

Ingredients

1 1/4 Lbs Ham steak

1/4 Cup black coffee

2 Tsps Bacon fat

2 Tbsps Butter

1/4 Cup Water

1 Tbsp Ketchup

Method

1.   Let ham steak come to temperature for 20 minutes. Blot it with a dry paper towel, so it browns and doesn't steam in the pan.

2.   Heat the olive oil in a skillet over medium flame.

3.   Add ham in heated oil and cook for seven minutes from both sides.

4.   Transfer the brown color cooked ham to the plate.

5.   Add water and coffee in the same skillet and cook over a low flame with constant stirring.

6.   Stir in ketchup and butter and cook for one minute.

7.   Pour the sauce over ham and serve.

18   Filet Mignon Steak Pizzaiola

Servings: 2 | **Time**: 40 mins | **Difficulty:** Medium

Nutrients per serving: Calories: 580 kcal | Fat: 42g | Carbohydrates: 8.8g | Protein: 40g | Fiber: 1.6g

Ingredients

Filet Mignon Steaks:

Salt to taste

2 Steaks Filet Mignon

Black pepper to taste

1 Tbsp Olive oil

Peppers and Mushrooms

Red Sauce:

2 Tbsp Dry white wine

1 Tbsp Olive oil

1/2 sliced green bell pepper

4 oz Sliced mushrooms

1/2 sliced Red bell pepper

1/4 Cup sliced Onion

1/4 Tsp thyme leaves Butter (Garlic Parmesan)

2 oz Butter

1/4 Tsp grated Raw garlic

2 oz grated Parmesan cheese

1/2 Cup Rao's Arrabiatta Sauce

Method

1. Keep steaks at room temperature.

2. Rub salt, oil, and pepper over the surface of filet mignon and set aside.

3. Add butter, cheese, and garlic in a bowl and toss well.

4. Transfer the mixture to cling film. Roll the film and give a log shape to it. Place the cling film with butter mixture in the fridge until further use.

5. Heat olive oil in a pan over medium flame.

6. Add steaks in heated oil and sear for three minutes.

7. Now place the pan in the oven at 375 °F and cook until steaks are done.

8. Transfer the steaks into the plate and cover to keep them warm.

9. Again heat olive oil in the same pan over medium flame.

10. Add bell peppers and onion and cook for five minutes with occasional stirring.

11. Sprinkle thyme and toss.

12.   Remove the pan from the flame and transfer the veggies to the plate. Set aside.

13.   Now add red sauce to a pan and lightly warm it up.

14.   Pour the sauce into the serving plate and place the steak over it.

15.   Pour the butter cheese mixture over the steaks, and at the end, top steaks with stirred fried veggies.

16.   Serve.

19   Instant Pot Vegetable Beef Soup

Servings: 6 | **Time**: 1 hr 20 mins | **Difficulty**: Easy

Nutrients per serving: Calories: 321 kcal | Fat: 14.87g | Carbohydrates: 10g | Protein: 32.83g | Fiber: 2.5g

Ingredients

1 1/2 Lbs cubed beef chuck

6 oz diced Turnip

1 Tbsp Olive oil

5 oz sliced Celery

4 oz cut String beans

4 oz sliced Carrots

3 oz diced Onions

32 oz beef broth

Two sliced Garlic cloves

Salt to taste

1/2 Cup red wine

2 Tsps beef base

2 Tbsps tomato paste

1 Tbsp mushroom powder

2 Tsps gelatin powder

Two bay leaves

4 Tbsps butter

Two whole cloves

1/2 Tsp rubbed dried marjoram

1 Tsp rubbed dried thyme

Black pepper to taste

Method

1. Heat the pan over medium flame and add beef to it.

2. Cook beef until it gets brown.

3. Transfer the beef into the pressure cooker with 4 tbsps beef broth.

4. Now add all the remaining ingredients to the cooker and mix well.

5. Cover the pressure cooker and shift it to soup mode.

6. When beef is done, add in marjoram and thyme and mix.

7. Sprinkle salt and pepper to adjust the taste.

8. Serve and enjoy it.

20   Low Carb Beef Stroganoff

Servings: 4 | **Time:** 30 mins | **Difficulty:** Medium

Nutrients per serving: Calories: 466 kcal | Fat: 36.6g | Carbohydrates: 5.86g | Protein: 26.5g | Fiber: 0.4g

Ingredients

2 oz Philadelphia Cream Cheese

1 Lb ground Beef, lean

1/4 Cup sliced Onions

4 oz sliced Mushrooms

3 Tbsps Butter

1 Tbsp Worcestershire sauce

2 Tbsps Brandy

Black pepper to taste

1 Tsp Beef base

1 Cup sour cream

1 Tbsp chopped parsley

1 1/2 pinches grated Nutmeg

Salt to taste

Method

1.   First, cook cauliflower rice in heated oil over medium flame for a few minutes.

2.   When the cauliflower rice is done, transfer them to a bowl and cover them to keep them warm.

3.   Heat olive oil in a skillet and sauté mushrooms for five minutes with occasional stirring.

4.   Add some more butter and stir in onions.

5.   Cook onions for few minutes and then transfer onions and mushrooms into the plate.

6.   Now, add ground beef in the same pan and cook it while breaking it with a spoon for a few minutes.

7.   Pour in Worcestershire sauce and toss well.

8.   Stir in beef base and brandy.

9.   In the end, add mushroom mixture and spread nutmegs.

10.   Let it simmer for a few minutes.

11.   Mix in cream cheese and cook to melt it.

12.   Then add sour cream and let it simmer.

13.   When the sauce gets thicken, sprinkle parsley, salt, and black pepper and toss well.

14.   Serve and enjoy it.

21 Pulled Pork Keto Stuffed Mushrooms

Servings: 2 | **Time:** 50 mins | **Difficulty**: Medium

Nutrients per serving: Calories: 548 kcal | Fat: 41g | Carbohydrates: 6.7g | Protein: 39.3g | Fiber: 1.4g

Ingredients

1/2 Cup keto coleslaw

2 Portobello mushroom caps

1 Cup shredded Cheddar cheese

1 Cup pulled Pork

1/4 Cup BBQ sauce Optional for the Mushroom Caps:

2 Tbsps Italian Dressing

1 Tbsp Olive oil

Method

1.   Lightly warm the pulled pork and add it to a bowl.

2.   Add cheese, salt, BQQ sauce, and black pepper.

3.   Now, make a small cavity in the center of the mushroom cap and fill it with a pulled pork mixture.

4.   Arrange the stuffed mushroom caps in a baking tray sprayed with oil and lined with parchment paper.

5.   Bake in a preheated oven at 400 degrees for 35 minutes.

6.   Spread coleslaw over baked mushroom caps.

7.   Serve and enjoy it.

22 Homemade Sloppy Joe Hot Pockets

Servings: 6 | **Time**: 35 mins | **Difficulty:** Medium

Nutrients per serving: Calories: 379 kcal | Fat: 28.5g | Carbohydrates: 8g | Protein: 23g | Fiber: 3g

Ingredients

2 Cups Sloppy Joe Filling

Hot Pocket Dough

1 1/2 Cups shredded Mozzarella cheese

1 Egg, beaten

2 oz Cream cheese

1 1/3 Cups Almond flour

1/4 Tsp Baking soda

3 Tbsps Whey protein powder

Method

1.   Add mozzarella cheese and cream cheese in a bowl and microwave the bowl for three minutes to melt the cheese. Whisk them well.

2.   Crack an egg in the cheese mixture and mix.

3.   Stir in almond flour, baking soda, and protein powder.

4.   Mix to combine everything well. Keep the dough aside for 30 minutes.

5.   Now roll out the dough between butter paper sprayed with oil.

6.   Spread the dough with the butter paper in a baking tray.

Assembly:

1.   Slice the dough in the required size and number.

2.   Spread sloppy joe filling at the center of each slice of the dough.

3.   Fold the dough and press the edges gently.

4.   Bake in a preheated oven at 400 degrees for 20 minutes.

5.   Serve and enjoy it.

23   Juicy Smoked Chicken Leg Quarters

Servings: 4 | **Time:** 2 hrs 10 mins | **Difficulty:** Difficult

Nutrients per serving: Calories: 261 kcal | Fat: 21g | Carbohydrates: 1.5g | Protein: 16g | Fiber: 0.1g

Ingredients

Four sliced Chicken leg

1 Tbsp Olive oil

3 Tsp Dry Rub for Chicken

Salt to taste

Smoker Pellets

signature blend, pecan

Method

1.   Dry chicken leg quarters with a paper towel. Remove any extra pieces of fat from the back of the chicken.

2.   Mix chicken rub and oil in a small bowl.

3.   Brush the chicken with oil mixture and set aside for one hour.

4.   Preheated the grill on smoke mode.

5.   Place the chicken over a preheated grill and let it cook on smoke mode for one hour.

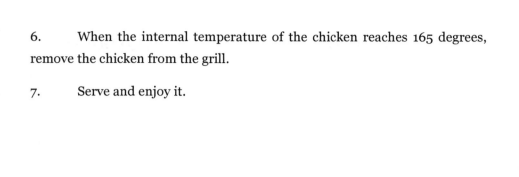

6.   When the internal temperature of the chicken reaches 165 degrees, remove the chicken from the grill.

7.   Serve and enjoy it.

24   Italian Sausage, Peppers and Onions with Sauce

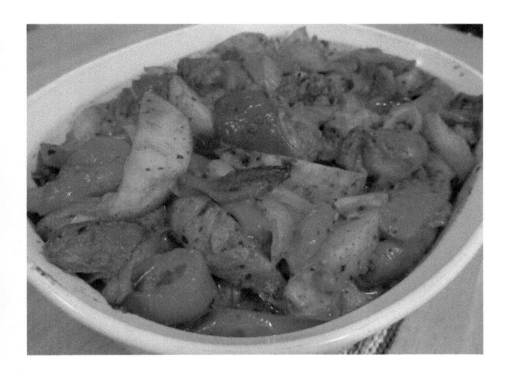

Servings: 4 | **Time:** 30 mins | **Difficulty**: Medium

Nutrients per serving: Calories: 420 kcal | Fat: 32.5g | Carbohydrates: 8g | Protein: 23.5g | Fiber: 1.5g

Ingredients

1 Lb Italian sausage

2 oz sliced Onion

9 oz sliced Bell pepper, any one color or mix

Salt to taste

1 Tbsp Olive oil

1/2 Cup Rao's Marinara Sauce

1 Tsp minced garlic

Black pepper to taste

Method

1.   Add sliced onions, sausage, oil, and pepper in a bowl.

2.   Transfer the mixture to a baking tray.

3.   Bake in a preheated oven at 400 degrees for 40 minutes.

4.   After 40 minutes, remove the pan from the oven and pour in marinara sauce.

5.   Serve and enjoy it.

25 Smoked Beer Can Chicken with Dry Rub

Servings: 4 | **Time**: 1 hr 25 mins | **Difficulty**: Difficult

Nutrients per serving: Calories: 337 kcal | Fat: 18g | Carbohydrates: 1.3g | Protein: 36g

Ingredients

1 Tbsps oil

One whole Chicken

3 Tbsps Chicken Rub

2 Cups Beer

Method

1.   Remove the chicken bits from the cavity. Dry the chicken well with paper towels.

2.   Mix oil and chicken rub in a small bowl.

3.   Brush the oil mixture over the whole surface of the chicken.

4.   Add 2 cups of beer to the chicken throne.

5.   Mix in two spoons of chicken rub into the liquid.

6.   Put the chicken throne in the chicken's cavity. Chicken should stand stable over the chicken throne.

7.   Place the chicken with the chicken throne over the pan.

8.   Cook, bake, or grill the chicken, whatever you want, for one hour till the chicken's central temperature reaches 16 degrees.

9.   Remove the chicken from the chicken throne.

10.   Slice the chicken and serve.

26 Creamy Keto Mac and Cheese with Ham

Servings: 4 | **Time:** 25 mins | **Difficulty**: Medium

Nutrients per serving: Calories: 404 kcal | Fat: 60g | Carbohydrates: 7g | Protein: 13g | Fiber: 7g

Ingredients

1 Lb Cauliflower

Three slices Bacon

10 oz cubed Ham

1/4 Cup Onion

1 Tsp Chicken Base

1 Tsp Garlic

1/4 Cup dry White wine

2 oz Cream cheese

1/4 Tsp White pepper

1/4 Cup Water

1/2 Cup Mozzarella cheese

1 Tsp Worcestershire sauce

1 Cup Cheddar cheese

Method

1. Steam the chopped cauliflower until they get soft and wilt.

2. Transfer cauliflower in a bowl and set aside.

3. Cook bacon in a skillet over medium flame until bacon becomes crispy; it will take seven minutes.

4. Transfer the bacon to the plate and leave the bacon fat in the pan.

5. Add garlic and onion to the same pan and cook for three minutes.

6. After three minutes, pour water and wine. Mix.

7. Add cream cheese and chicken base. Stir and cook until cheese melts.

8. Now add mozzarella cheese, white pepper, cheddar cheese, and Worcestershire.

9. Let it simmer for seven minutes.

10. When the sauce gets a little thick, add ham and steamed cauliflower into the pan and toss gently.

11. Place bacon at the top and serve.

27 Easy Sausage and Cabbage Dinner

Servings: 4 | **Time:** 30 mins | **Difficulty:** Medium

Nutrients per serving: Calories: 306 kcal | Fat: 21g | Carbohydrates: 8.5g | Protein: 20g | Fiber: 2g

Ingredients

1 Lb Italian sausages

Four strips Raw bacon

1 Lb sliced cabbage

2 oz sliced onion

Salt to taste

One chopped Garlic clove

Black pepper to taste

Method

1. Now, preheat the grill.

2. Place sausage over the heated grill and cook for few minutes or until they are done.

3. Now cook bacon in heated oil in a pan until they become crispy.

4. Mix garlic and onions and cook for five minutes.

5.   Add chopped cabbage and cook until it gets soft.

6.   Add cabbage in batches to cook them properly.

7.   In the end, add sliced grilled sausage, pepper, and salt to the pan and toss well.

8.   Serve and enjoy it.

28 Baja Fish Tacos with Chipotle Lime Crema

Servings: 4 | **Time**: 20 mins | **Difficulty:** Easy

Nutrients per serving: Calories: 524 kcal | Fat: 42g | Carbohydrates: 11.5g | Protein: 27g | Fiber: 4g

Ingredients

BAJA FISH TACOS:

2 Tbsp Avocado oil

1 Lb Halibut

Black pepper to taste Tortillas

Sea salt to taste

Simple Red Cabbage Slaw

1 Tsp Sea salt

1/2 shredded red cabbage

One diced Jalapeño

1/2 Red sliced onion

2 Tbsps of Lime juice

CHIPOTLE LIME CREMA:

1/2 Cup Plain yogurt

1/2 Tsp Sea salt

1/4 Tsp Chipotle powder

1/4 Tsp Garlic powder

1 Tbsp Lime juice

TOPPINGS:

1/2 Cup chopped Cilantro

Two sliced Jalapeños

One diced avocado, diced

2 Tbsps lime wedges

Method

1.   Rub fish with salt and pepper and set aside for a while.

2.   Whisk all the ingredients of red cabbage slaw in a bowl.

3.   Mix them using hands, do message to thoroughly mix them. Keep it aside.

4.   In another bowl, mix all the items of chipotle lime crema and place the bowl in the fridge for a while. The chipotle lime crema is ready

5.   Heat oil in a pan over medium flame.

6.   Add fish and cook for five minutes from both sides.

7.   Transfer the cooked fish strips to a plate and set them aside.

8.   Lightly toast the tortillas in a pan.

9.   Place fish strips over each tortilla followed by cabbage slaw, jalapeno slices, sprinkle cilantro, place avocado, and at the end spread chipotle lime crema.

29 Spinach Artichoke Pizza

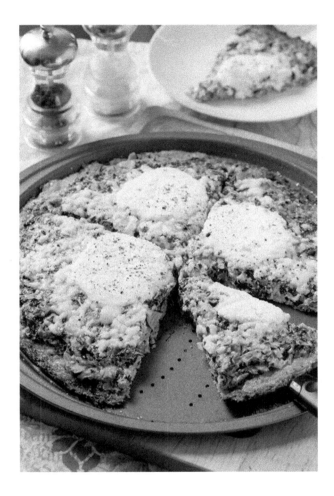

Servings: 4 | **Time**: 40 mins | **Difficulty**: Medium

Nutrients per serving: Calories: 366 kcal | Fat: 28g | Carbohydrates: 8g | Protein: 22g | Fiber: 3g

Ingredients

Fathead Pizza Crust

1/4 Cup Almond flour

1 1/2 Cup grated Mozzarella cheese

1 Egg

2 oz Cream cheese

2 Tbsps Whey protein powder

Spinach Artichoke Dip

1/4 Tsp White pepper

4 oz Cream cheese

8 oz Spinach

1 Cup Shredded Jack cheese

1 Tsp Red wine vinegar

8 Cups artichoke hearts

1/4 Cup chopped Onion

1 tbsp butter

1 Tsp minced Garlic

Additional Cheese

1 Tbsp mayonnaise

1/2 cup Monterey Jack Cheese

Method

1.   Combine cream cheese and mozzarella cheese in a bowl and microwave them for half a minute to melt them.

2.   Crack an egg in a cheese mixture and mix.

3.   Stir in protein powder and almond flour and toss well to mix everything.

4.   Knead the dough a little.

5.   Now roll the dough between butter paper and spread it in a pan.

6.   Cook the dough in a preheated oven at 400 degrees for about 15 minutes.

7.   Melt the butter in a skillet over medium flame and sauté garlic and onions in heated butter for two minutes.

8.   Mix in artichokes and spinach and mix.

9.   Pour red wine and add pepper and salt.

10.   Add mayonnaise and mix. The dipping is ready.

11.   Spread jack cheese over the baked crust and then spread artichoke dipping over the curst. toppings.

12.   Place the pan in the oven again for a few minutes to lightly melt and warm the

13.   Serve and enjoy it.

30 White Chicken Enchiladas

Servings: 8 | **Time**: 40 mins | **Difficulty:** Medium

Nutrients per serving: Calories: 433 kcal | Fat: 33g | Carbohydrates: 3g | Protein: 30g | Fiber: 0.5g

Ingredients

Eight crepes

Chicken Enchilada Filling

Salt to taste

1 Lb shredded Rotisserie chicken

Black pepper to taste

White Cheese Sauce

1/4 Tsp Salt

2 Cups grated Monterey Jack cheese

4 oz diced Green chills

4 oz Cream cheese

1/2 Tsp White pepper

1 1/2 Tsp ground Cumin

1/2 Tsp granulated Onion powder

1/2 Tsp granulated Garlic powder

Method

1.   Mix salt and pepper with shredded chicken.

2.   Heat the skillet over medium flame.

3.   Add all the items of sauce into the pan and cook until they melt with occasional stirring.

4.   Bring it to simmer for a few minutes to thicken the sauce.

5.   When required, consistency of the sauce is achieved, then remove the pan from the flame.

6.   Spread half of the sauce over a casserole tray sprayed with oil.

7.   Now spread chicken mixture over the tortilla ad roll them up.

8.   Place the rolled tortilla in a casserole with the seamed side facing downwards.

9.   Spread the remaining sauce over the tortilla and bake in a preheated oven at 350 degrees for 30 minutes.

10.   Serve and enjoy it.

31 Mexican Cornbread Casserole Taco Pie

Servings: 8 | **Time:** 45 mins | **Difficulty**: Medium

Nutrients per serving: Calories: 436 kcal | Fat: 30g | Carbohydrates: 8g | Protein: 31g | Fiber: 3g

Ingredients

Ground Beef Taco Meat

2 Tbsps Tomato paste

1 Lb Ground beef

Salt to taste

2 Tbsps Taco seasoning

Black pepper to taste

1 Cup Cheddar cheese

1/2 Cup Beef broth

"Cornbread" Base

1 Cup grated Mozzarella Cheese

2 Cups Almond flour

2 oz Cream cheese

3 Eggs

1 Tbsp Baking powder

1/4 Tsp Sweet Corn Extract

Method

1.   Cook ground beef in a pan over medium flame.

2.   Use a spoon to break the beef while cooking.

3.   After ten minutes, add taco seasoning, beef broth, and tomato paste. Cook for few minutes until liquid is reduced to half.

4.   Sprinkle salt, cheese, and pepper. Remove the pan from the flame.

5.   Blend eggs, extract, cheese, baking powder, and almond flour in a processor to form a thick batter.

6.   Transfer the batter to a pan sprayed with oil and spread it evenly.

7.   Spread taco meat over the batter.

8.   Bake in a preheated oven at 30 degrees for 40 minutes.

9.   Spread cheese and bake again to melt the cheese.

10.   Serve and enjoy it.

32   Chicken Pizza Crust

Servings: 4 | **Time:** 40 mins | **Difficulty**: Medium

Nutrients per serving: Calories: 222 kcal | Fat: 11g | Carbohydrates: 1g | Protein: 30g

Ingredients

1 Cup grated Mozzarella cheese

1 Lb shredded chicken breast

Salt to taste

2 Eggs

Black pepper to taste

Method

1.   Add shredded chicken, pepper, and salt in a bowl. Toss well.

2.   Add all the remaining ingredients and mix them using your hands.

3.   Transfer the mixture over a baking tray lined with parchment paper.

4.   Bake in a preheated oven at 400 degrees for 20 minutes.

5.   Spread the desired toppings over the baked pizza and place them in the oven again.

6.   Bake the pizza for 12 minutes.

7.   Serve and enjoy it.

33 Low Carb Mexican Chicken Casserole

Servings: 8 | **Time:** 55 mins | **Difficulty:** Medium

Nutrients per serving: Calories: 184 kcal | Fat: 11g | Carbohydrates: 8g | Protein: 12g | Fiber: 2g

Ingredients

1 1/4 Cups Enchilada sauce

6 Cups cooked cauliflower rice

1 Egg

2 cups cooked and shredded Chicken

2 cups grated Mexican Blend Cheese

4 oz diced Green chilies

1/4 Tsp Salt

1 Tsp Ground cumin

Optional Toppings:

Diced Avocado

Extra enchilada sauce

Diced Tomatoes

Sour cream

Cilantro

Method

1.   Mix cauliflower, cheese, chilies, salt, egg, and cumin in a bowl. Set aside.

2.   Spread cauliflower rice over the casserole tray sprayed with oil. Press the rice firmly.

3.   Bake the casserole in a preheated oven for 35 minutes.

4.   Mix enchilada sauce and meat in a bowl.

5.   Spread the meat mixture over cauliflower rice and add cheese.

6.   Bake again for ten minutes to melt the cheese.

7.   Serve and enjoy it.

34   Low Carb Taco Salad

Servings: 4 | **Time:** 25 mins | **Difficulty**: Medium

Nutrients per serving: Calories: 530 kcal | Fat: 42g | Carbohydrates: 9g | Protein: 32g | Fiber: 5g

Ingredients

Black pepper to taste

1 Lb Ground beef

One cubed Avocado

Two chopped Romaine hearts

4 oz cubed Cheddar cheese

Salt to taste

2 Tbsps sliced Red onion

3 oz Grape tomatoes

1 Tsp Ground cumin

Mexican Vinaigrette

1 Cup Cilantro Lime Vinaigrette

Optional Ingredients:

Sour cream Salsa

Method

1.   Cook beef in a pan over medium flame for ten minutes and use a spoon to break it while cooking.

2.   Stir in salt, cumin, and pepper.

3.   Add taco seasoning and cook for one minute.

4.   Prepare the vinaigrette by following the instructions written in the packet.

5.   Transfer all the ingredients, including the cooked beef, to a bowl.

6.   Pour in the dressing over the mixture in the bowl and toss well.

7.   Spread salsa and cream and serve.

35 Ground Beef Taco

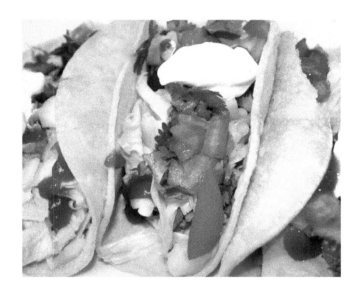

Servings: 6 | **Time:** 25 mins | **Difficulty**: Medium

Nutrients per serving: Calories: 432 kcal | Fat: 33g | Carbohydrates: 7g | Protein: 28g | Fiber: 2g

Ingredients

Ground Beef Taco Meat

One recipe Taco Seasoning

1 Lb Ground beef

2 Tbsps Tomato paste

Salt to taste

1/2 Cup Beef broth

Pepper to taste

Taco Shells

6 Cheese Taco Shells

1/2 Cup Salsa

2 Cups chopped Lettuce

1/2 Cup shredded Cheese

1/4 Cup Mined Purple onion

One sliced Avocado

1/2 Cup Sour cream

1/4 Cup chopped Cilantro

Method

1.   Add lemon juice and avocado in a bowl and set aside until further use.

2.   Cook ground beef in a pan over medium flame with constant stirring to break the beef during cooking.

3.   Add taco seasoning and cook for two minutes.

4.   Stir in beef broth and let it simmer for few minutes.

5.   Sprinkle salt and pepper according to the taste.

6.   Spread the taco meat in taco cheese shells and add toppings according to your taste.

36   Herb Roasted Chicken

Servings: 6 | **Time:** 2 hrs 45 mins | **Difficulty**: Difficult

Nutrients per serving: Calories: 409 kcal | Fat: 30g | Carbohydrates: 2g | Protein: 30g

Ingredients

1 Tbsp Avocado oil

Salt to taste

One whole Chicken

Black pepper to taste

Compound Butter

2 Tsps chopped Parsley

4 Tbsps Butter

1 Tsp shredded lemon zest

Ingredients for Chicken Cavity and Pan:

Two crushed Garlic cloves

One chopped Onion

1/2 Cup Water

One whole Lemon

Parsley sprigs as required

Method

1.   Combine lemon zest, butter, lemon juice, and parsley in a bowl.

2.   Rub the butter mixture over the chicken pieces to coat them well.

3.   Then rub lemon, salt, olive oil, and pepper over the chicken pieces

4.   Preheat oven to 350 degrees F and position rack to the middle of the oven.

5.   Fill the chicken cavity with lemon, garlic, and parsley.

6.   Place the chicken in a pan and spread onion, parsley, garlic, and lemon around the chicken.

7.   Then roast the chicken in a preheated oven at 350 degrees for 100 minutes.

8.   You can add water when the pan starts getting dry during roasting.

9.   Transfer the chicken onto the plate.

10.   Serve and enjoy it.

37   Keto Beef Stew

Servings: 6 | **Time:** 2 hrs 30 mins | **Difficulty:** Difficult

Nutrients per serving: Calories: 288 kcal | Fat: 20g | Carbohydrates: 8g | Protein: 20g | Fiber: 2g

Ingredients

6 oz chopped Celery root

1 1/4 Lbs cubed Beef chuck roast

Two sliced Celery ribs

8 oz chopped whole mushrooms

4 oz sliced Pearl onions

Two sliced Garlic cloves

Black pepper to taste

3 oz sliced Carrot

2 Tbsps Tomato paste

5 Cups Beef broth

2 Tbsps Olive oil

1 Bay leaf

Salt to taste

1/2 Tsp Dried thyme

Method

1.   Rub beef with the oil and set aside.

2.   Heat the oil in a heavy bottom pan over medium flame.

3.   Sauté mushrooms in heated oil for two minutes.

4.   Transfer the cooked mushrooms to the bowl where other veggies are added.

5.   Again heat the olive oil over medium flame in the same pot.

6.   Cook beef in heated oil for a few minutes.

7.   Add tomato paste, thyme, and bay leaf and toss well.

8.   Cook for two minutes.

9.   Slowly pour in broth with constant stirring.

10.   Let it simmer for two minutes.

11.   Cover the pot and let it cook for 90 minutes over low flame.

12.   When beef is done, add veggies and mix well.

13.   Simmer for five minutes over medium flame

14.   Cover the pot and cook for 40 minutes over low flame.

15.   Sprinkle salt and pepper to adjust the flavor.

16.   Serve and enjoy it.

38 Bacon Wrapped Pork Chops with Apple Cider Vinegar Glaze

Servings: 4 | **Time:** 25 mins | **Difficulty**: Medium

Nutrients per serving: Calories: 358 kcal | Fat: 24g | Carbohydrates: 1.5g | Protein: 32.5g

Ingredients

Pork Chops

Four slices Bacon

1 1/4 Lbs boneless Pork chops

1 Tbsp Olive oil

Black pepper to taste

Salt to taste

Apple Cider Vinegar Glaze

1/2 Cup Water

1/4 Cup diced Onion

1 Tsp Chicken base

Two minced Garlic cloves

1/4 Cup Apple cider vinegar

2 Tbsps Butter

3 Sprigs of thyme

1 Tsp sugar

Method

1. Rub pork chops with salt, oil, and pepper and set aside.

2. Heat olive oil in a skillet over medium flame.

3. Add pork chops and cook from both sides for five minutes.

4. Transfer the chops into the plate and cover to keep them warm.

5. Now sauté garlic and onions for two minutes.

6. Stir in thyme and chicken base—Cook for one minute.

7. Add vinegar and water and mix well.

8. Cook until half of the sauce is evaporated.

9. Add butter and cook to mix it with the sauce.

10. Let it simmer for a few minutes.

11. At this point, you can adjust the taste by adding salt and pepper.

12. Pour the sauce over pork and serve.

39   Hamburger Steak and Gravy

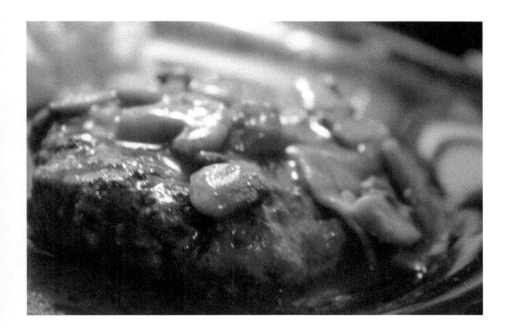

Servings: 4 | **Time**: 25 mins | **Difficulty**: Medium

Nutrients per serving: Calories: 612 kcal | Fat: 52g | Carbohydrates: 5g | Protein: 29g | Fiber: 1g

Ingredients

Hamburger Steaks

2 Tsps Montreal Steak Seasoning

1 1/4 Lbs Ground beef

2 Tsps Worcestershire sauce

1 Tbsp minced Parsley

1 Tsp Oil

1/4 Cup crushed Pork rinds

Salt to taste

1/4 Cup Heavy cream

Black pepper to taste

Mushroom and Onion Gravy

1/4 Cup Water

1/4 Cup diced Onions

1 Tsp Beef base

8 oz sliced Mushrooms

2 Tbsps Whisky

1/3 Cup Heavy cream

1 Tbsp Butter

Method

1.   Soak pork rinds in cream for ten minutes. The panade is ready. Set aside.

2.   Combine beef, soaked pork rinds, steak seasoning, Worcestershire, and parsley. Use your hands to mix all the ingredients evenly.

3. Make patties of the required size out of the mixture.

4. Season the patties with salt and pepper.

5. Heat olive oil in a skillet over medium flame.

6. Cook patties in heated oil for five minutes from both sides.

7. Transfer cooked patties (hamburger steak) into the plate and set aside.

8. Now melt butter in the same pan and sauté mushrooms for two minutes with constant stirring.

9. Add onion and stir. Cover the pan and cook for two minutes.

10. Stir in the beef base, whisky, and water.

11. Mix in heavy cream and stir well.

12. Let it simmer until the sauce gets thickens.

13. Add butter and salt and pepper to adjust the flavor.

14. Pour the sauce over the patties and serve.

40 Easy Pan-Seared Lamb Chops with Mustard Cream Sauce

Servings: 4 | **Time:** 30 mins | **Difficulty:** Medium

Nutrients per serving: Calories: 426 kcal | Fat: 30g | Carbohydrates: 4g | Protein: 31g

Ingredients

Pan-Seared Lamb Chops

1 Tbsp chopped Rosemary

1 1/2 Lbs Lamb chops

Salt to taste

Two crushed Garlic cloves

2 Tbsps Olive oil

Black pepper to taste

Mustard Cream Pan Sauce

2 Tbsps Brandy

1 Tbsp minced Shallot Sprig of Rosemary

1 Tbsp grainy Mustard

1/2 Cup Beef broth

2/3 Cup Heavy cream

2 Tsps Worcestershire sauce

Salt to taste

2 Tsps Lemon juice

1 Tsp Erythritol Sprig of Thyme

2 tbsps Butter

Black pepper to taste

Method

1.   Add garlic, rosemary, lamb chops, and olive oil in a bowl and toss well.

2.   Place chops in a baking tray and sprinkle salt, pepper, and rosemary mixture.

3.   Cover the tray and place in the fridge for several hours.

4.   Heat olive oil in a skillet over medium flame.

5.   Add chops and cook for eight minutes.

6.   Change the side of the chops and cook the other side for seven minutes.

7.   Transfer the cooked lamb chops to a plate and set aside.

8.   Sauté shallots in a pan over a low flame.

9.   Pour in brandy and beef broth.

10.   Increase the flame to medium and let it simmer for one minute.

11.   Now add mustard, erythritol, and Worcestershire and toss well.

12.   Add rosemary, cream, and thyme and simmer for ten minutes.

13.   Squeeze lime juice and add butter. Toss and simmer until desired consistency is achieved—the mustard cream sauce is ready.

14.   Pour the sauce over lamb chops; serve and enjoy it.

41   Low Carb Pork Stir Fry

Servings: 4 | **Time:** 15 mins | **Difficulty:** Easy

Nutrients per serving: Calories: 226 kcal | Fat: 12g | Carbohydrates: 10g | Protein: 19g | Fiber: 4g

Ingredients

1 Tbsp minced Ginger

3/4 Lb stripped Pork loin

12 oz Broccoli florets

1 Tbsp Extra dry sherry

2 Tbsps Avocado

1 Tsp minced Garlic

1 Cup Green onions

1 Tsp cornstarch

One sliced Red bell pepper

2 Tbsps Tamari soy sauce

1 1/2 Tbsps sugar

1 Tsp sesame oil

Optional Ingredients:

Sesame seeds

Red pepper flakes

Method

1.   Combine minced garlic, ginger, pork loin, and oil in a mixing bowl.

2.   Now add chopped bell pepper, sliced onions, chopped broccoli in layer form in bowl.

3.   Mix in cornstarch and sweetener. Toss well.

4.   Then add sesame oil, soy sauce, and sherry and mix.

5.   Heat olive oil in a wok over medium flame.

6.   Add pork and cook for a few minutes without touching it.

7.   Cook from both sides, and when they are completely cooked, transfer them to the plate.

8.   Now shift the veggies into the wok and cover the wok.

9.   Cook for one minute.

10.   Add pork and mix well.

11.   Mix in the sauce and let it boil with occasional stirring for one minute.

12.   When the sauce gets thickens, remove the wok from the flame.

13.   Serve and enjoy it.

42   Low Carb Malibu Chicken

Servings: 4 | **Time:** 50 mins | **Difficulty:** Medium

Nutrients per serving: Calories: 696 kcal | Fat: 55g | Carbohydrates: 4g | Protein: 46g

Ingredients

Salt to taste

4 Chicken breasts

Black pepper to taste

Malibu Dipping Sauce

3 Tbsps Yellow mustard

1/2 Cup Mayonnaise

1 Tbsp powdered sugar

Crumb Topping

2 Tsps Granulated garlic

3/4 Cup crushed Pork rinds

3/4 Cup grated Parmesan cheese

1/4 Tsp Salt

1 Tsp granulated Onion

1/8 Tsp Pepper

Top With

4 oz Swiss cheese

Eight pieces of sliced Deli ham

Method

1.   First, add pork rinds in a food processor and crush them.

2.   Transfer the crushed pork rinds to a bowl and set aside.

3.   Rub dry chicken with salt and pepper and set aside.

4.   Whisk mustard, mayonnaise, and sweetener in a bowl.

5.   Pour less than half of the mayo mixture over the chicken and reserve the remaining for further use.

6.   Toss to evenly coat the chicken with the mayo mixture and place it in the fridge for two hours to marinate.

7.   Now, in another bowl, combine seasoning, cheese, and pork rinds.

8.   Spread half of the mixture in a baking tray.

9.   Place the chicken in the tray and spread the other half of the mixture on the chicken pieces' top.

10.   Bake in a preheated oven at 350 degrees for 40 minutes until the chicken is done.

11.   Sprinkle ham and cheese and bake again to melt the cheese.

12.   Serve and enjoy it.

43 Grilled Buffalo Shrimp Tacos with Blue Cheese Crema

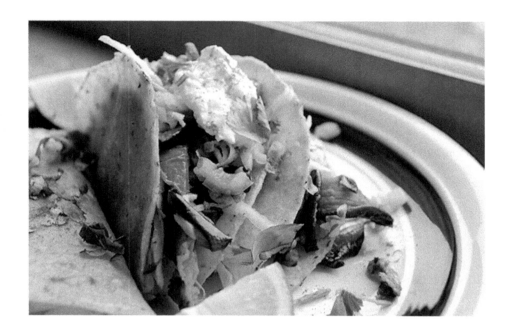

Servings: 4 | **Time:** 30 mins | **Difficulty**: Medium

Nutrients per serving: Calories: 188 kcal | Fat: 18g | Carbohydrates: 6g | Protein: 2g | Fiber: 3g

Ingredients

GRILLED BUFFALO SHRIMP TACOS:

2 Tbsps Lime juice

1 Lb Shrimp

½ diced Red onion

1 Cup Hot Sauce

1/4 Cup Avocado oil

12 Corn tortillas

SIMPLE RED CABBAGE SLAW:

One diced Jalapeño

1/2 chopped Red cabbage

½ Red sliced onion

1 Tsp Sea salt

3   Tbsps lime juice

BLUE CHEESE CREMA:

1 Tbsp Lime juice

1 Cup Greek yogurt

1/2 Tsp Sea salt

2 oz crumbled Blue cheese Coldwater as required

TOPPINGS:

One diced Avocado

1 Cup chopped Cilantro

2 Tbsps Lime wedges

Two sliced Jalapeños

Method

1. Whisk lime juice, onions, hot sauce, and avocado oil in a bowl.

2. Add shrimps and mix well to evenly coat the shrimps.

3. Place the bowl in the fridge for two hours to marinate the shrimps.

4. Combine jalapeno, lime juice, red cabbage, onion, and salt in a bowl and mix well.

5. Message all the ingredients using hands to soften the cabbage.

6. The red cabbage slaw is ready. Set aside.

7. Mix yogurt, lime juice, salt, and blue cheese in a mixing bowl.

8. Pour in water and transfer the mixture to a blender and blend to get a smooth mixture.

9. You can add more water to get the desired consistency.

10. Lightly toast the tortillas over a preheated grill for half a minute.

11. Now place the shrimps over the grill sprayed with oil.

12. Grill shrimps for three minutes from both sides.

13. Spread cabbage slaw over tortillas, place cilantro, jalapeno, shrimp, blue cheese crema, and avocado.

14. Serve with hot sauce and enjoy it.

44   Cream of Mushroom Pork Chops

Servings: 4 | **Time:** 30 mins | **Difficulty:** Easy

Nutrients per serving: Calories: 483 kcal | Fat: 40g | Carbohydrates: 6g | Protein: 21g | Fiber: 1g

Ingredients

Four thin, bone-in pork chops

2 1/2 tbsp divided avocado oil

1 pound mushrooms, sliced

1 tbsp minced onion

One clove minced garlic

1/3 cup chicken broth unsalted

1/3 cup dry white wine

1/8 tsp powdered dried sage

1/2 cup heavy cream

salt & pepper

1/4 tsp chopped fresh thyme leaves

Method

1.   Let the chops of pork stand for at least 20 min at room temp. This guarantees that they cook equally & don't get rough. With around 2 tsp of oil, rub all sides of the pork & sprinkle with salt. Chop the onion & garlic, then cut the thyme. In a shallow bowl, put the wine & chicken broth along.

2.   On med-high heat, heat a wide skillet. Once hot, put 2 to 3 teaspoons of Oil or sufficiently for the skillet's bottom to swirl & coat. Once the surface shimmers, the oil is hot. In the pan, Put the chops of pork & lower the heat to med. Cook on each side for around 3 1/3 mins. Take it from the plate & cover with foil.

3.   In the skillet, pour one tablespoon of oil & swirl to coat. Put the mushrooms as the oil shimmers, then stir to coat—Cook for two mins undisturbed. Mix the mushrooms & put the garlic & onions in the skillet. 1 min to cook & stir. Cook for the extra min. Then scrape all the brown bits from the skillet's bottom with the wine & chicken broth. Let it boil & decrease by half.

4.   Cook till the sauce thickens & put the powdered sage, fresh thyme & heavy cream (this is a thinner sauce). (this is a thinner sauce). Sprinkle with salt.

5.   Put the pork chops in the skillet & carry them to the plate or place the pork chops on the mushrooms & sauce and eat.

45 Indian Chicken Tikka Wings

Servings: 4 | **Time:** 40 mins | **Difficulty**: Easy

Nutrients per serving: Calories: 396 kcal | Fat: 33g | Carbohydrates: 2g | Protein: 23g

Ingredients

Ten whole chicken wings Tikka Marinade

1 cup coconut milk full fat

1 1/2 tbsp ground cilantro

2 tsp ground chili pepper

1 1/4 tsp salt

1/2 chopped cilantro

Three cloves chopped garlic

1/4 cup fresh juice of the lemon

Citrus Cilantro Sauce

1/4 cup fresh juice of a lemon

1/4 cup coconut milk full fat

1/8 tsp salt

1/2 bunch coriander

1-2 tbsp erythritol

Method

1.   Preparation: Split the wings into wings & drums with a fine knife. Throw away the tips or reserve them for soup. Mix the ingredients in a big plastic zip-lock bag for your Tikka Chicken marinade & put the wings. For 24 to 48 hrs, marinate.

2.   Roast the Wings: Take the Tikka Chicken wings back from the marinade & blot with paper towels. Sprinkle with salt. Make the grill preheat. Oil the barbecue grill & cook the wings - around ten min each side - till cooked through.

3.   Sauce: Mix the ingredients for your sauce in a processor when the wings are frying, & blend. Uh, taste.

4.   Take the chicken tikka wings from the barbecue & either spill over the sauce & serve or place it on the side with the sauce.

5.   Oven Method: Put & spread the chicken wings on the sheet skillet. Bake for 30-40 mins at 350 & finish for a few mins more under the broiler till the wings have a good color on them.

46   Low Carb City Chicken

Servings: 4 | **Time:** 25 mins | **Difficulty**: Easy

Nutrients per serving: Calories: 300 kcal | Fat: 16.93g | Carbohydrates: 2.84g | Protein: 33g | Fiber: 1.2g

Ingredients

salt & pepper

1 pound boneless pork loin

One big egg

2 tbsp divided olive oil

Low Carb Coating Gluten Free

1/4 cup Parmesan Cheese

1/2 cup almond flour

1 tbsp minced parsley

1/4 tsp pepper

1/2 tsp salt

1/4 tsp garlic powder, coarse

1/4 tsp onion powder, granulated

Eight wooden skewers

Method

1.   Break the pork into cubes of around 1 inch. Onto Eight skewers, string the pork. With salt & pepper, season.

2.   In a jar big enough to accommodate a whole skewer, combine the ingredients to coat.

3.   On a broad dinner plate, put the threaded skewers. Break the egg and spill the pork over it. Switch each of the skewers that are covered in the egg.

4.   Heat a med skillet on med heat to cook or saute. Apply one tablespoon of oil when hot & swirl to cover the plate.

5.   Take the skewer of the pork, allowing any excess egg to drain back onto the plate, & roll it into the breading combination. Ensure that it is properly coated. Put it in the skillet. Three more skewers, repeat the same process.

6.   Fry the City Chicken on either side for around 1 1/2 mins, on all four sides. Remove & cook the leftover skewers of City Chicken on a paper towel. Serve at room temp.

47   Peri Peri Chicken

Servings: 4 | **Time:** 4 hrs 45 mins | **Difficulty:** Easy

Nutrients per serving: Calories: 520 kcal | Fat: 44g | Carbohydrates: 8g | Protein: 27g | Fiber: 4g

Ingredients

2 cups divided Peri-Peri sauce

4 Chicken quarters

Method

1.   Before putting them in the freezer bag with one cup of Peri-Peri sauce, drizzle the chicken thighs with   one tsp of salt. For Four hours or overnight, seal & put in the freezer to marinate.

2.   Oven preheated to210 degrees C.

3.   Pull off the extra marinade & cut the marinated chicken from the frozen bag.

4.   In a shallow bowl, put ½ cup of the Peri-Peri sauce.

5.   In a broad casserole bowl or on a cookie sheet, put the chicken parts & bake for 20 to 30 mins. As the chicken cooks, baste this with the peri-peri sauce you put in the bowl every 10 mins.

6.   Serve on the side with the leftover 1/2 cup Peri-Peri sauce.

48   Easy Keto Pad Thai

Servings: 2 | **Time**: 23 mins | **Difficulty:** Easy

Nutrients per serving: Calories: 300 kcal | Fat: 22g | Carbohydrates: 13g | Protein: 13g | Fiber: 4g

Ingredients

2 tbsp Rice wine vinegar

2 tbsp Fish sauce

1 tbsp Lime juice

1 tbsp Granulated artificial sweetener, we used Splenda

Two big Eggs

2 tbsp Peanut oil

2 tsp minced garlic

14 ounces spiralized courgette

Four chopped Scallions

5 ounces Bean sprouts

2 tbsp finely chopped Fresh Coriander

4 tsp minced peanuts

Method

1.   In a tiny saucepan, mix fish sauce, rice vinegar, artificial sweetener & lime juice, then carry to a simmer on med-high heat.

2.   Fry the eggs in a tiny cup. Place the egg on the boiling sauce & whisk the full time. Let the eggs boil   till they are finished. Take it from the heat.

3.   Sauté the peanut oil & garlic for 1 min in a pan on med-high heat. Stir in the scallions.

4.   Put the scallions & courgette and finish cooking for 1 min.

5.   Over the courgette, spill the sauce & put the bean sprouts. Sauté and after this take it from the heat.

6.   Add the coriander & peanuts to the garnish. Immediately serve.

49 Air Fryer Pork Chops

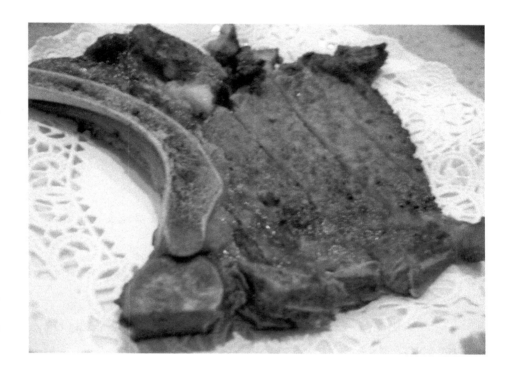

Servings: 4 | **Time:** 14 mins | **Difficulty:** Easy

Nutrients per serving: Calories: 248 kcal | Fat: 13g | Carbohydrates: 2g | Protein: 29g | Fiber: 1g

Ingredients

4 Boneless pork chops

1 tbsp Olive oil

2 tsp Garlic powder

2 tsp Onion powder

Two tsp Paprika

1 tsp Salt

1/2 tsp Pepper

Method

1.　　Mix the onion powder, garlic powder, paprika & salt in a shallow bowl.

2.　　Use a thin layer of olive oil to brush the chops of pork & then rub the spice mix onto them.

3.　　Put the chops of pork in the basket of the airy fryer, operating in batches. Put the pork chops side-by-side.

4.　　Set the temp to 185 degrees C for 9 mins. Begin cooking the chops with the pork.

5.　　Stop the timer halfway through & remove the basket, tossing the pork chops over. Remove the basket as well as the timer begins.

50 Instant Pot Roast Beef

Servings: 6 | **Time:** 1 hr. 17 mins | **Difficulty:** Easy

Nutrients per serving: Calories: 473 kcal | Fat: 29g | Carbohydrates: 5g | Protein: 45g | Fiber: 1g

Ingredients

3 pounds Chuck roast

2 tsp Italian seasoning

2 tsp Garlic powder

2 tsp Onion powder

1 tsp Kosher salt

1 tbsp Olive oil

One roughly chopped Carrot

½ roughly chopped Onion

Two crushed cloves Garlic

1 tbsp Tomato paste

5 cup Red wine

1 tbsp Worcestershire

2 cups Beef broth

Method

1.   Slice the chuck roast into pieces of 1 pound.

2.   Mix the onion powder, Italian Seasoning, Kosher salt & garlic powder in a tiny bowl.

3.   Rub it over the beef with the seasoning combination.

4.   Set SAUTE as your Instant Pot & add olive oil. Put in the pot brown on either side for 2 mins with   the seasoned chuck roast bits. Remove & set aside the browned beef.

5.   Leave the saute for the Instant Pot. Put the red wine, then simmer for five mins.

6.   Whisk together the red wine & put the tomato paste, Worcestershire & beef broth in the pot.

7.   With the onion, garlic & carrots, put your browned beef in the liquid in a pot.

8.   Secure the lid input and placed SEALING on the valve. For 40 mins, set to HIGH Intensity.

9.   Click CANCEL whenever the timer goes off & let it release the natural pressure release for ten min. Transfer the valve to VENTING after ten min to relieve the excess pressure.

10.   Set aside & extract the cooked beef from a liquid. For the veggies to be removed, strain the liquid into a fine-mesh strainer.

Lightning Source UK Ltd.
Milton Keynes UK
UKHW021845040521
383144UK00003B/360